EFFORTLESS
KETO

50 Very Quick & Easy Ketogenic Recipes

ANNA MARIE QUEEN

TABLE OF CONTENTS

BREAKFAST

1 – Eggs with Spinach and Cheese

Preparation	Cooking	Servings
10 min	**25 min**	**6**

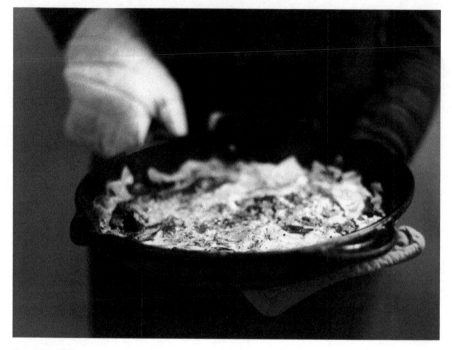

Ingredients

- 6 whole eggs
- 4 oz cottage cheese
- 3-4 oz chopped spinach 1/4 cup parmesan cheese 1/2 cup of milk

Direction

1. Preheat your oven to 375°F/190°C.

2. In a large bowl, whisk the eggs, cottage cheese, parmesan, and milk.
3. Mix in the spinach.
4. Transfer to a small, greased oven dish.
5. Sprinkle the cheese on top.
6. Bake for 25-30 minutes.
7. Let cool for 5 minutes and serve.
8. Serve!

Per Serving: Calories: 190 Fat: 24g Carbohydrates: 2.3g Protein: 15.3g

2 – Juicy Scotch Egg

Preparation	Cooking	Servings
15 min	**28 min**	**6**

Ingredients

- 6 large eggs
- 2 package beef Sausage (12 oz)
- 10 slices thick-cut beef bacon
- 6 toothpicks

Direction

1. Hard-boil the eggs, peel the shells, and let them cool.

2. Slice the sausage into four parts and place each part into a large circle.
3. Put an egg into each circle and wrap it in the sausage.
4. Place inside your refrigerator for 1 hour.
5. Make a cross with two pieces of thick-cut bacon.
6. Place a wrapped egg in the center, fold the bacon over the top of the egg and secure with a toothpick.
7. Cook inside your oven at 450°F/230°C for 25 minutes.
8. Enjoy!

Per Serving: Calories: 325 Fat: 25.3g Carbohydrates: 1.6g Protein: 17.3g

3 – Toasty Cauliflower

Preparation	Cooking	Servings
12 min	**8 min**	**6**

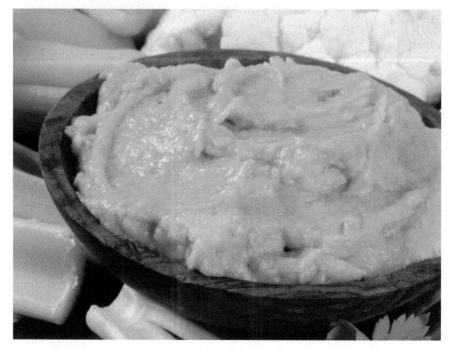

Ingredients

- 2 large egg
- 2 grated cauliflower head
- 2 chopped avocado
- 1 cup shredded mozzarella cheese
- Salt & Black pepper

Direction

1. Set the oven to preheat at 420 F, then line the baking tray with a parchment paper
2. Cook the cauliflower in the microwave on high for 7 minutes
3. Allow the cauliflower to cool, then drain on a paper towel.
4. Remove the excess moisture by pressing with a clean kitchen towel, then put them in a bowl.
5. Add the egg and mozzarella, then stir
6. Add the seasonings and mix evenly, then shape the mixture into medium squares
7. Arrange the squares on the prepared baking tray.
8. Allow baking until browned evenly, for about 20 minutes
9. In the meantime, puree the avocado with black pepper and salt.
10. Top with the pureed avocado.
11. Serve!

Per Serving: Calories: 126Fat: 7gCarbohydrates: 10gProtein: 10g

4 - Crepes Avocado Egg

Preparation	Cooking	Servings
12 min	6 min	6

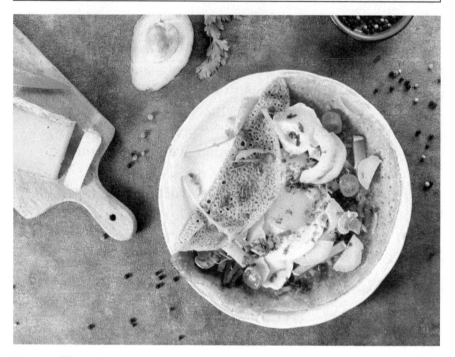

Ingredients

- 6 eggs
- 1 sliced avocado
- 3 teaspoons olive oil
- 1 cup alfalfa sprouts
- 6 slices shredded turkey breast

Direction

1. Pour the olive oil into a pan and heat over medium heat

2. Crush the eggs and cook for 3 minutes on each side of the pan as you spread to cook evenly.
3. Remove the eggs from heat, then top with avocado, turkey breast, sprouts, and alfalfa, then roll up well.
4. Serve!

Per Serving: Calories: 361 Fat: 24.2g Carbohydrates: 14.2g Protein: 26.3g

5 - Shallots With Spinach and Bacon

Preparation	Cooking	Servings
12 min	22 min	6

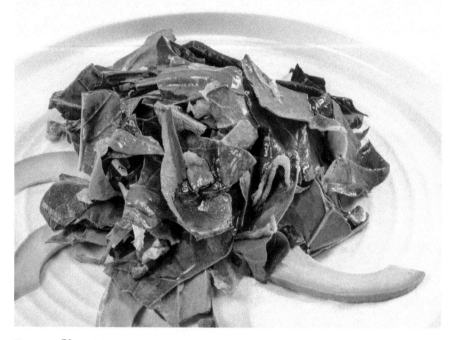

Ingredients

- 18 oz raw spinach
- 1 cup chopped white onion
- 1 cup chopped shallot
- 2 pound raw bacon slices
- 3 tbsp butter

Direction

1. Slice the bacon strips into small narrow pieces.

2. In a skillet, heat the butter and add the chopped onion, shallots, and bacon.
3. Saute for 15-20 minutes or until the onions start to caramelize and the bacon is cooked.
4. Add the spinach and saute on medium heat. Stir frequently to ensure the leaves touch the skillet while cooking.
5. Cover and steam for around 5 minutes, stir and continue until wilted.
6. Serve!

Per Serving: Calories: 140 Fat: 12.5g Carbohydrates: 5.2g Protein: 4.8g

APPETIZERS AND SNACKS

6 - Eggplant Fries

Preparation	Cooking	Servings
15 min	**20 min**	**6**

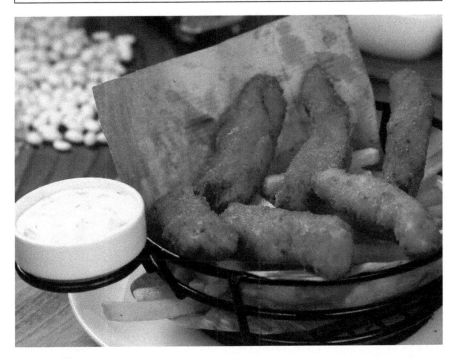

Ingredients

- 4 whole eggs
- 3 cups almond flour
- 3 tablespoons coconut oil, spray
- 3 eggplant, peeled and cut thinly
- Salt and pepper to taste

Direction

1. Preheat your oven to 400 degrees Fahrenheit.

2. Take a bowl and mix with salt and black pepper in it.

3. Take another bowl and beat eggs until frothy.

4. Dip the eggplant pieces into eggs.

5. Then coat them with a flour mixture.

6. Add another layer of flour and egg.

7. Then, take a baking sheet and grease with coconut oil on top.

8. Bake for about 15 minutes.

9. Serve and enjoy!

Per Serving: Calories: 245 Fat: 14.2g Carbohydrates: 3.9g Protein: 6.2g

7 - Avocado Stuffed Parmesan

Preparation	Cooking	Servings
15 min	**20 min**	**6**

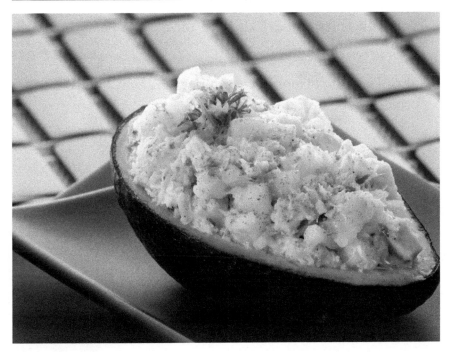

Ingredients

- 1 whole avocado
- 1 tablespoon chipotle sauce
- 1 tablespoon lime juice
- ¼ cup parmesan cheese
- Salt and pepper to taste

Direction

1. Prepare avocado by slicing half lengthwise and discard the seed.

2. Gently prick the skin of the avocado with a fork.

3. Set your avocado halves, skin down on the small baking sheet lined with aluminum foil.

4. Top with sauce and drizzle lime juice.

5. Season with salt and pepper.

6. Sprinkle half parmesan cheese in each cavity, set your broiler to high for 2 minutes.

7. Add rest of the cheese and return to your broiler until cheese melts and avocado slightly browns.

8. Serve hot and enjoy!

Per Serving: Calories: 31 Fat: 40.2g Carbohydrates: 7.3g Protein: 5.2g

8 - Creamsicles Coco and Orange

Preparation	Cooking	Servings
15 min	**0 min**	**6**

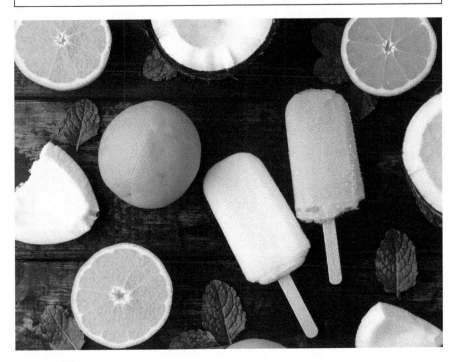

Ingredients

- 1 cup of coconut oil
- 1 cup heavy whipping cream
- 6 ounces cream cheese
- 2 teaspoon orange mix
- 12 drops liquid stevia

Direction

1. Add the listed ingredients to a bowl.

2. Use an immersion blender and blend the mixture well.

3. Take a silicone tray and add the mixture.

4. Keep in the refrigerator for 2-3 hours.

5. Serve and enjoy!

Per Serving: Calories: 155 Fat: 21g Carbohydrates: 0.6g Protein: 0.9g

9 - Popsicles Coffee

Preparation	Cooking	Servings
15 min	**0 min**	**6**

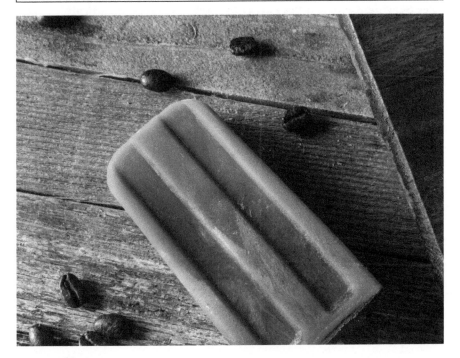

Ingredients

- 3 tablespoons chocolate chips, sugar-free
- 3 cups coffee, brewed and cold
- 4 cup heavy whip cream
- 3 teaspoons natural sweetener

Direction

1. Blend in heavy whip cream, sweetened, and coffee in your blender.

2. Mix them well.

3. Pour the mix into popsicle molds.

4. Add a few chocolate chips.

5. Keep in the fridge for 2 hours.

6. Serve and enjoy!

Per Serving: Calories: 125 Fat: 11.2g Carbohydrates: 2.2g Protein: 2.3g

10 - Popsicles Berry

Preparation	Cooking	Servings
15 min	**0 min**	**6**

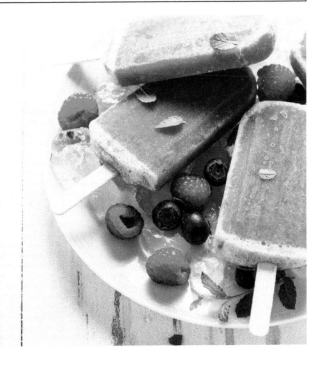

Ingredients

- 1 cup mixed blackberries and blueberries
- 3 cups coconut cream
- 3 teaspoons stevia

Direction

1. Blend the listed ingredients into your blender.

2. Blend until smooth.

3. Pour the mix into popsicle molds.

4. Keep in the fridge for 2 hours.

5. Serve and enjoy!

Per Serving: Calories: 154 Fat: 16.2g Carbohydrates: 3.1g Protein: 1.3g

11 - Scrambled Pesto Eggs

Preparation	Cooking	Servings
10 min	**7 min**	**6**

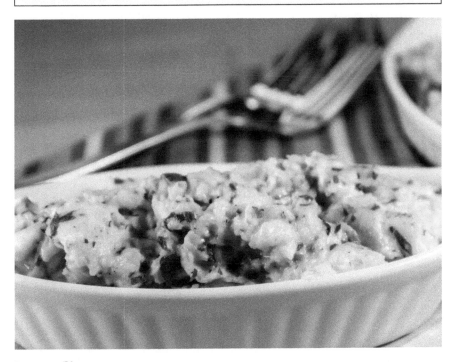

Ingredients

- 4 large whole eggs
- 2 tablespoon butter
- 2 tablespoon pesto
- 4 tablespoons creamed coconut milk
- Salt and pepper as needed

Direction

1. Take a bowl and crack open your egg

2. Season with a pinch of salt and pepper
3. Pour eggs into a pan
4. Add butter and introduce heat
5. Cook on low heat and gently add pesto
6. Once the egg is cooked and scrambled, remove heat
7. Spoon in coconut cream and mix well
8. Turn on the heat and cook on LOW for a while until you have a creamy texture
9. Serve and enjoy!

Per Serving: Calories: 325 Fat: 35g Carbohydrates: 3.2g Protein: 18g

12 - Chicken Wings Black Berry

Preparation	Cooking	Servings
30 min	**60 min**	**6**

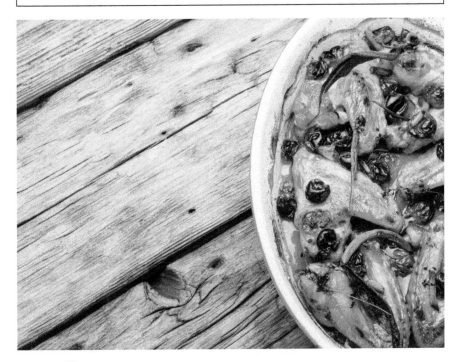

Ingredients

- 4 pounds chicken wings, about 20 pieces
- 1 cup blackberry chipotle jam
- Salt and pepper to taste
- 1 cup water

Direction

1. Add water and jam to a bowl and mix well

2. Place chicken wings in a zip bag and add two-thirds of the marinade

3. Season with salt and pepper

4. Let it marinate for 30 minutes

5. Pre-heat your oven to 400 degrees F

6. Prepare a baking sheet and wire rack, place chicken wings in the wire rack and bake for 15 minutes

7. Brush remaining marinade and bake for 30 minutes more

8. Enjoy!

Per Serving: Calories: 455 Fat: 36g Carbohydrates: 2g Protein: 33g

BEEF

13 - Beef Meatballs

Preparation	Cooking	Servings
15 min	20 min	6

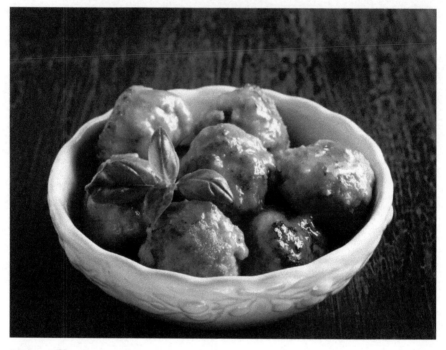

Ingredients

- 2 lb ground beef
- 1 cup grated parmesan cheese
- 2 tbsp minced garlic (or paste)
- 1 cup mozzarella cheese
- 1 tsp freshly ground pepper

Direction

1. Preheat your oven to 400°F/200°C.

2. In a bowl, mix all the ingredients together.
3. Roll the meat mixture into 6 generous meatballs.
4. Bake inside your oven at 170°F/80°C for about 18 minutes.
5. Serve with sauce!

Per Serving: Calories: 377 Fat: 21g Carbohydrates: 1.8g Protein: 16g

14 - Beef Casserole

Preparation	Cooking	Servings
15 min	**35 min**	**6**

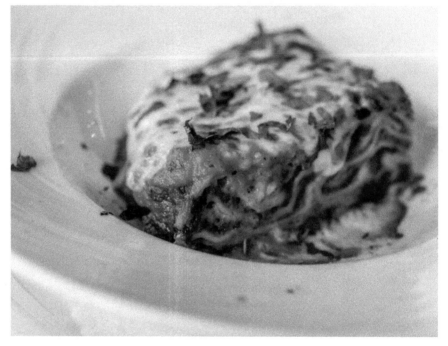

Ingredients

- 1 lb. ground beef
- 1 cup chopped onion
- 1 bag coleslaw mix
- 2 cups tomato sauce
- 2 tbsp lemon juice

Direction

1. In a skillet, cook the ground beef until browned and to the side.
2. Mix in the onion and cabbage to the skillet and sauté until soft.
3. Add the ground beef back in along with the tomato sauce and lemon juice.
4. Bring the mixture to a boil, then cover and simmer for 30 minutes.
5. Enjoy!

Per Serving: Calories: 265 Fat: 21g Carbohydrates: 6.2g Protein: 21g

15 - Ground Beef Hamburger Patties

Preparation	Cooking	Servings
15 min	12 min	6

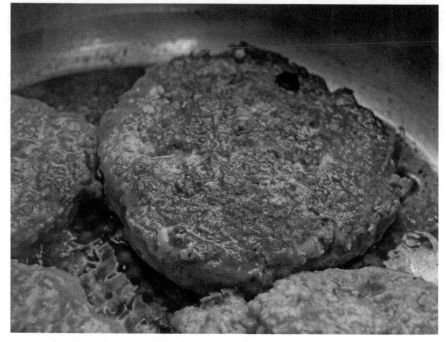

Ingredients

- 1 egg
- 12 oz. ground beef
- 2 oz. crumbled feta cheese
- 1 oz. butter
- Salt & Black pepper

Direction

1. In a mixing bowl, add the feta cheese, ground beef, black pepper, egg, and salt, then mix to combine well.
2. Shape the mixture into equal patties.
3. Put a pan on fire to melt the butter.
4. Cook the patties for 4 minutes on each side on medium-low heat.
5. Serve!

Per Serving: Calories: 445 Fat: 24g Carbohydrates: 2.2g Protein: 57g

PORK

16 - Pork Chops Onion and Bacon

Preparation	Cooking	Servings
15 min	50 min	6

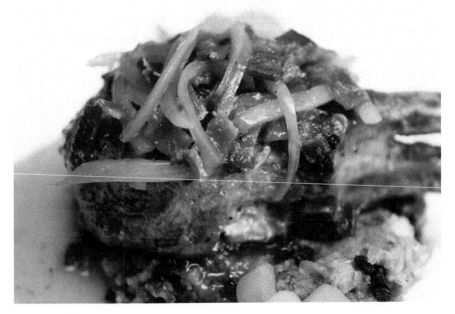

Ingredients

- 3 onions, peeled and chopped
- 6 bacon slices, chopped
- 1 cup chicken stock
- Salt and pepper to taste
- 6 pork chops

Direction

1. Heat up pan over medium-heat and add bacon

2. Stir and cook until crispy

3. Transfer to bowl

4. Return pan to medium heat and add onions, season with salt and pepper

5. Stir and cook for 15 minutes

6. Transfer to same bowl with bacon

7. Return the pan to heat (medium-high) and add pork chops

8. Season with salt and pepper and brown for 3 minutes

9. Flip and lower heat to medium

10. Cook for 7 minutes more

11. Add stock and stir cook for 2 minutes

12. Return the bacon and onions to the pan and stir cook for 1 minute

13. Serve and enjoy!

Per Serving: Calories: 315 Fat: 17g Carbohydrates: 6.2g Protein: 35g

17 - Medi Pork Classical

Preparation	Cooking	Servings
15 min	**30 min**	**6**

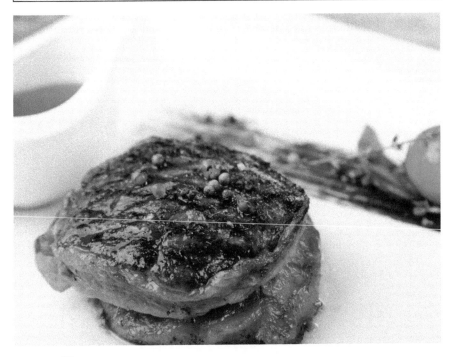

Ingredients

- 6 pork chops, bone-in
- Salt and pepper to taste
- 2 teaspoon dried rosemary
- 4 garlic cloves, peeled and minced

Direction

1. Season pork chops with salt and pepper
2. Place in roasting pan

3. Add rosemary, garlic in pan
4. Pre-heat your oven to 425-degree F
5. Bake for 10 minutes
6. Lower heat to 350-degree F
7. Roast for 25 minutes more
8. Slice pork and divide on plates
9. Drizzle pan juice all over
10. Serve and enjoy!

Per Serving Calories: 145 Fat: 2.2g Carbohydrates: 2.1g Protein: 25g

POULTRY

18 - Burn Fried Chicken

Preparation	Cooking	Servings
15 min	25 min	6

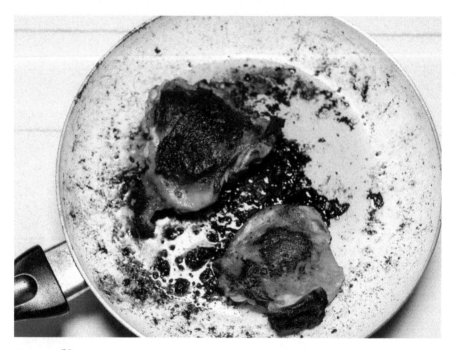

Ingredients

- 1 teaspoon cayenne pepper
- 1 teaspoon onion powder
- 1 teaspoon black pepper
- 3 teaspoons paprika
- 1 teaspoon ground thyme
- 1 teaspoon cumin
- 1/2 teaspoon salt

- 4 (12-ounce / 480-g) skinless, boneless chicken breasts
- 2 teaspoons olive oil

Direction

1. Mix the cayenne pepper, onion powder, black pepper, paprika, thyme, cumin, and salt in a bowl.
2. Rub the chicken breasts with the olive oil, then put it in the spice mixture. Make sure they are coated all around with the spices, then set aside to marinate for 5 minutes.
3. Preheat the air fryer to 375°F (190°C).
4. Put the chicken in the air fryer basket and cook for 10 minutes. Flip it over and cook for another 10 minutes.
5. Remove the chicken from the basket to a plate and let it rest for 5 minutes before serving.

Per Serving Calories: 454 Fat: 13g Carbohydrates: 2g Protein: 75g

19 - Chicken Taco Wings

Preparation	Cooking	Servings
15 min	15 min	6

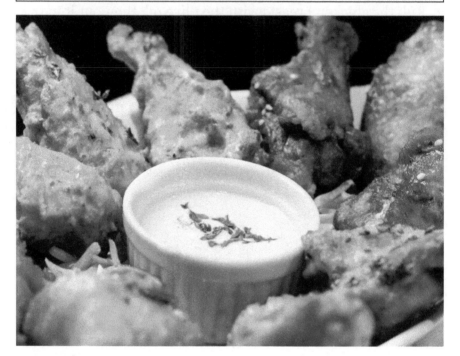

Ingredients

- 4 pounds chicken wings
- 2 tablespoon taco seasoning mix
- 3 teaspoons olive oil

Direction

1. Put the chicken wings in a Ziploc bag, then add the taco seasoning and olive oil.

2. Seal the bag and shake well until the chicken is coated thoroughly.

3. Preheat the air fryer to 350°F (180°C).

4. Put the chicken in the air fryer basket and cook for 6 minutes on each side until crispy.

5. Remove the chicken from the basket and serve on a plate.

Per Serving Calories: 344 Fat: 10g Carbohydrates: 2g Protein: 54g

20 - Tarragon Creamy Chicken

Preparation	Cooking	Servings
15 min	25 min	6

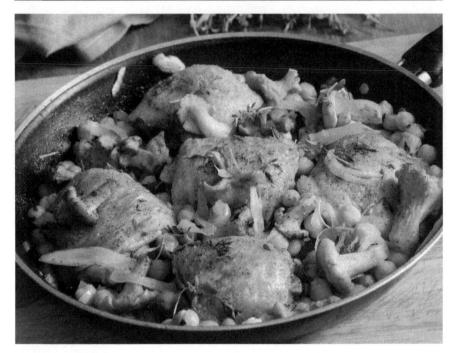

Ingredients

- 2 tablespoon butter
- 2 tablespoon olive oil
- 6 skinless, boneless chicken breasts
- Salt and fleshly ground black pepper, to taste 1/2 cup heavy cream
- 2 tablespoon Dijon mustard
- 3 teaspoons chopped fresh tarragon

Direction

1. Melt the butter in a pan over medium-high heat, then add the olive oil.
2. Season the chicken with salt and pepper then put it in the pan to fry for 15 minutes on both sides until the juices are clear. Remove them from the pan and set aside.
3. Pour the heavy cream in the pan and use a wooden spoon to scrape the parts stuck to the pan, then add the mustard and the tarragon. Mix well and let it simmer for 5 minutes.
4. Put the chicken back into the pan and cover it with the creamy sauce.
5. Serve the chicken drizzled with the sauce on a plate.

Per Serving Calories: 360 Fat: 17g Carbohydrates: 2.2g Protein: 52g

21 - Spicy Chicken Breast

Preparation	Cooking	Servings
15 min	10 min	6

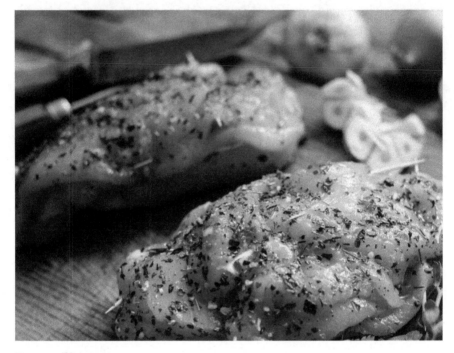

Ingredients

- 6 skinless, boneless chicken breast halves 1/8 cup extra virgin olive oil
- 1 lemon, juiced
- 3 teaspoons crushed garlic
- 1 teaspoon salt
- 2 teaspoons black pepper
- 1/2 teaspoon paprika
- 2 tablespoons olive oil, divided

Direction

1. Combine the olive oil, lemon, garlic, salt, pepper, and paprika in a bowl, then set aside.

2. Cut 3 slits into the chicken breasts to allow the marinade to soak in. Put the chicken in a separate bowl and pour the marinade over it.

3. Cover the bowl with plastic wrap and put in the refrigerator to marinate overnight.

4. Preheat the grill to medium heat and brush the grill grates with 1 tablespoon of olive oil.

5. Remove the chicken from the marinade and place it on the grill to cook for about 5 minutes until the juices are clear. Flip the chicken over and brush with the remaining olive oil. Grill for 3 minutes more.

6. Remove the chicken from the grill and serve on plates.

Per Serving Calories: 420 Fat: 21g Carbohydrates: 2.2g Protein: 54g

FISH

22 - Grilled Fish Salad

Preparation	Cooking	Servings
15 min	15 min	6

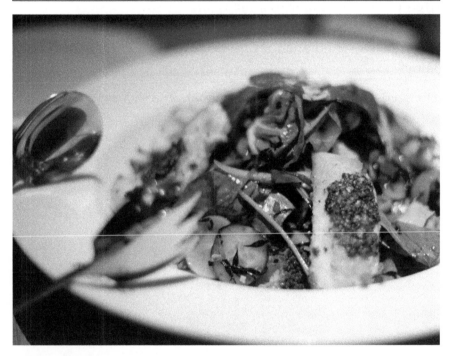

Ingredients

- 2 pound tuna fillet, skinless
- 2 white onion, sliced
- 1 teaspoon Dijon mustard
- 12 Nicoise olives, pitted and sliced
- 1/2 teaspoon anchovy paste

Direction

1. Brush the tuna with nonstick cooking oil; season with salt and freshly cracked black pepper. Then, grill your tuna on a lightly oiled rack for approximately 7 minutes, turning over once or twice.

2. Let the fish stand for 3 to 4 minutes and break into bite-sized pieces. Transfer to a nice salad bowl.

3. Toss the tuna pieces with the white onion, Dijon mustard, Nicoise olives, and anchovy paste. Serve well chilled, and enjoy!

Per Serving Calories: 124 Fat: 0.4g Carbohydrates: 3.4g Protein: 0.4g

23 - Cumin and Salmon Meal

Preparation	Cooking	Servings
15 min	5 min	6

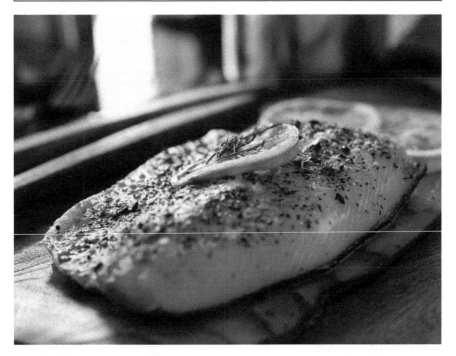

Ingredients

- 6 salmon fillets, boneless
- 2 tablespoon avocado oil
- 1 red onion, sliced
- 2 teaspoon chili powder
- 2 teaspoon cumin, ground

Direction

1. Heat up a pan with the oil over medium-high heat, add the onion and chili powder and cook for 2 minutes.
2. Add the fish, salt, pepper, and cumin, cook for 4 minutes on each side divide between plates and serve.

Per Serving Calories: 200 Fat: 12g Carbohydrates: 4g Protein: 15g

24 - Lemon Dill Trout

Preparation	Cooking	Servings
10 min	10 min	6

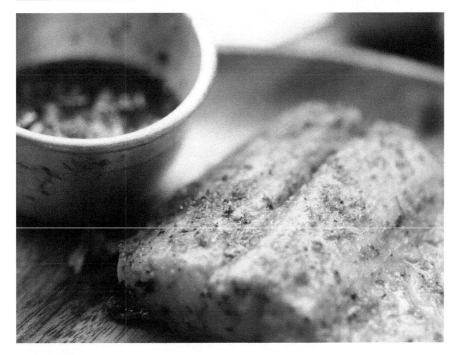

Ingredients

- 3 lb pan-dressed trout (or other small fish), fresh or frozen
- 2 tsp salt
- 1 cup butter or margarine
- 3 tbsp dill weed
- 4 tbsp lemon juice

Direction

1. Cut the fish lengthwise and season it with pepper.
2. Prepare a skillet by melting the butter and dill weed.
3. Fry the fish on high heat, flesh side down, for 2-3 minutes per side.
4. Remove the fish. Add the lemon juice to the butter and dill to create a sauce.
5. Serve the fish with the sauce.

Per Serving Calories: 455 Fat: 20g Carbohydrates: 1.2g Protein: 51g

SOUPS

25 - Zucchini Soup

Preparation	Cooking	Servings
15 min	**8 hours**	**8**

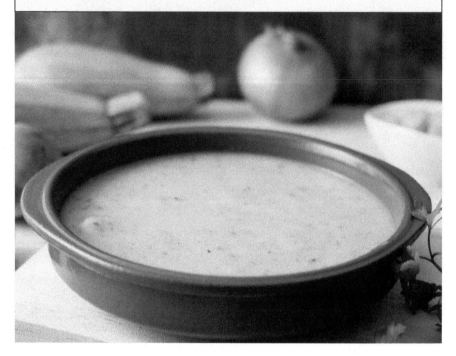

Ingredients

- 4 cups vegetable broth
- 4 zucchinis, cut in chunks
- 4 tablespoons sour cream, low fat
- 4 cloves garlic, minced
- Salt, pepper, thyme, and pepper, to taste

Direction

1. Add all the ingredients except sour cream to a crockpot.

2. Close the lid.

3. Cook for 6-8 hours on low.

4. Add sour cream.

5. Make a smooth puree by using a blender.

6. Serve hot with parmesan cheese if you want.

7. Enjoy!

Per Serving Calories: 70 Fat: 1.2g Carbohydrates: 8g Protein: 2.5g

26 - Soup with Poached Egg

Preparation	Cooking	Servings
15 min	15 min	6

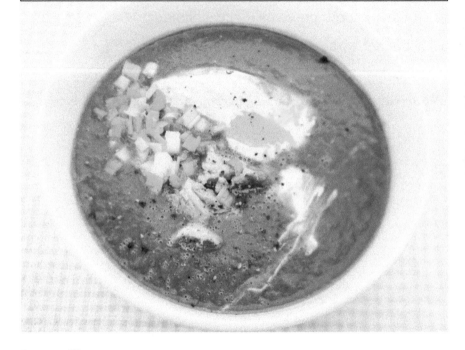

Ingredients

- 4 eggs
- 24 ounces chicken broth
- 2 head of romaine lettuce, chopped
- Salt, to taste

Direction

1. Bring the chicken broth to a boil.

2. Reduce the heat and poach the 2 eggs in the broth for 5 minutes.

3. Take two bowls and transfer the eggs into a separated bowl.

4. Add chopped romaine lettuce into the broth and cook for a few minutes.

5. Serve the broth with lettuce into the bowls.

6. Enjoy!

Per Serving Calories: 140 Fat: 5.1g Carbohydrates: 10g Protein: 15g

27 - Spanish Soup

Preparation	Cooking	Servings
20 min	6 min	6

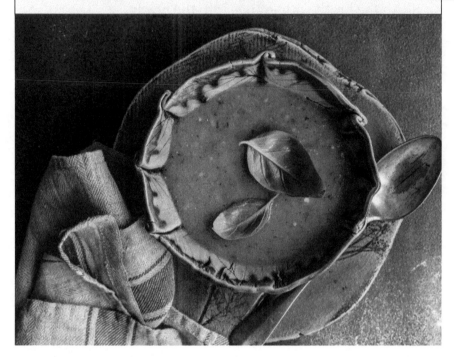

Ingredients

- 2 tomatoes, chopped

- 2 cucumber, peeled, seeded, and chopped

- 1 white onion, chopped

- 1 green bell pepper, seeded and chopped

- tablespoons olive oil, garlic-flavored

Direction

1 Add all the ingredients and mix them in a blender.

2 Blend until you get a smooth mixture.

3 Close the lid and cook for 5 minutes.

4 Let it refrigerate for 1 hour.

5 Garnish with bell pepper and chopped tomato.

6 Serve and enjoy!

Per Serving Calories: 123 Fat: 10g Carbohydrates: 8g Protein: 2.2g

28 - Butter Garlic Soup

Preparation	Cooking	Servings
15 min	7 min	6

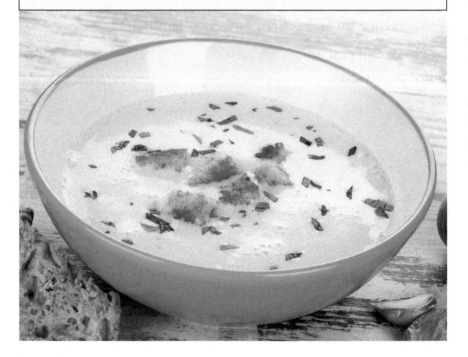

Ingredients

- 6 cups butternut squash, cubed
- 6 cups vegetable broth, stock
- ½ cup full-fat cream
- 3 garlic cloves, finely chopped
- Salt and pepper

Direction

1 Add butternut squash, garlic cloves, broth, salt, and pepper in a large pot.

2 Place the pot over medium heat and cover the lid.

3 Bring it to a boil, and then reduce the temperature.

4 Let it simmer for sometimes

5 Blend the soup for 1-2 minutes until you get a smooth mixture.

6 Stir the cream through the soup.

7 Serve and enjoy!

Per Serving Calories: 174 Fat: 12g Carbohydrates: 20g Protein: 3.2g

DESSERTS

29 – Low Carb Angel Cake

Preparation	Cooking	Servings
15 min	50 min	8

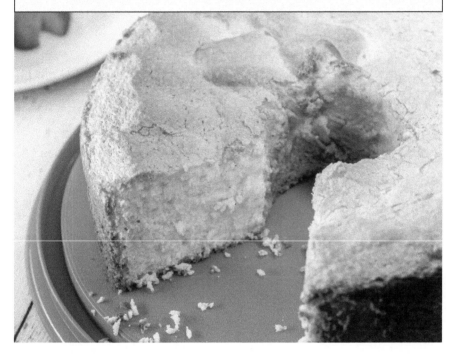

Ingredients

- 2 cup of Egg white powder

- 2 cup of powdered Erythritol

- 2 tsp of strawberry extract

- 16 egg whites

- 4 tsp cream of tartar

Direction

1. Pre-heat your oven to 350 degrees F
2. Sift in whey protein, confectioners Erythritol and mix together
3. Take a large bowl and whip in egg whites, a pinch of salt, and mix until you have a foamy mix
4. Add cream of tartar, keep beating until very stiff and add your desired flavor extract
5. Quick fold in whey mixture
6. Pour the mixture into a 10-inch tube pan (greased) and bake for 45 minutes
7. Serve and enjoy!

Per Serving Calories: 149 Fat: 3.2g Carbohydrates: 4g Protein: 1.9g

30 - Mini Cheesecake

Preparation	Cooking	Servings
3 hours	**40 min**	**8**

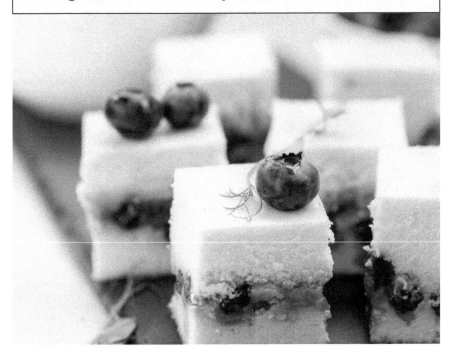

Ingredients

- 8 oz cream cheese
- 1/2 cup of sour cream
- 4 large whole eggs
- 1/2 c of natural sweetener
- 1/2 tsp of vanilla extract

Direction

1. Pre-heat your oven to 350 degrees F
2. Take a medium bowl and add cream cheese, sour cream, eggs, sweetener, vanilla and blend until thoroughly mixed
3. Place silicon liners in cups of a muffin tin
4. Pour the batter in your liners and bake for 30 minutes
5. Refrigerate for 3 hours
6. Serve and enjoy!

Per Serving Calories: 149 Fat: 14g Carbohydrates: 6g Protein: 2.2g

31 - Jalapeno and Bacon Fat Bomb

Preparation	Cooking	Servings
15 min	15 min	8

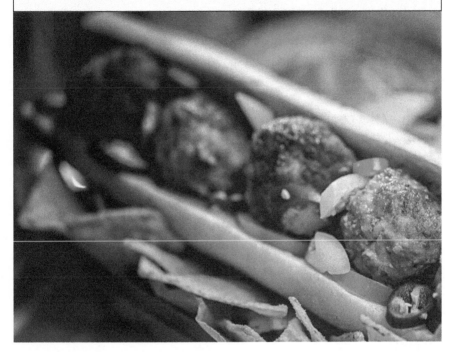

Ingredients

- 18 large jalapeno peppers
- 16 beef bacon strips
- 12 ounces full fat cream cheese
- 4 teaspoons garlic powder
- 2 teaspoon chili powder

Direction

1. Pre-heat your oven to 350 degrees Fahrenheit.

2. Place a wire rack over a roasting pan and keep it on the side.

3. Make a slit lengthways across jalapeno pepper and scrape out the seeds, discard them.

4. Place a nonstick skillet over high heat and add half of your bacon strip; cook until crispy.

5. Drain them.

6. Chop the cooked bacon strips and transfer them to a large bowl.

7. Add cream cheese and mix.

8. Season the cream cheese and bacon mixture with garlic and chili powder.

9. Mix well.

10.   Stuff the mix into the jalapeno peppers and wrap raw bacon strips all around.

11. Arrange the stuffed wrapped jalapeno on a prepared wire rack.

12. Roast for 10 minutes.

13. Transfer to a cooling rack and serve!

Per Serving Calories: 219 Fat: 11g Carbohydrates: 7.2g Protein: 11g

32 - Poppy Seeds Fat Bomb

Preparation	Cooking	Servings
60 min	**0 min**	**8**

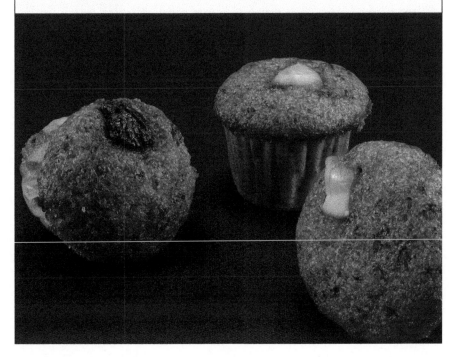

Ingredients

- 16 ounces cream cheese, soft

- 6 tablespoons erythritol

- 2 tablespoon poppy seeds

- 2 lemon zest

- 4 tablespoons lemon juice

- 8 tablespoons sour cream

Direction

1. Add listed ingredients to a bowl and mix using a hand mixer on low.

2. Once mixed, mix for 3 minutes on a medium-high setting.

3. Spoon mixture into mini cupcake cases and chill for 1 hour.

4. Enjoy once done!

    Per Serving Calories: 70 Fat: 0.5g Carbohydrates: 2.2g Protein: 1.1g

33 - Rich Choco Fat Bombs

Preparation	Cooking	Servings
3 hours	**0 min**	**8**

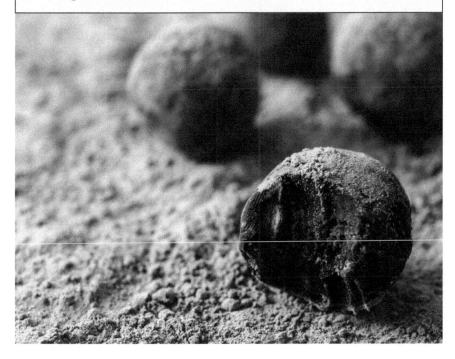

Ingredients

- 16 ounces cream cheese, soft

- 4 ounces icing mix

- 2 teaspoon vanilla essence

- 14 ounces heavy cream

- 10 ounces sugar-free chocolate

Direction

1. Take a heatproof bowl and add water; let it simmer. Take another bowl and add chocolate; place bowl in simmer water to melt the chocolate.

2. Take another bowl and add cream cheese, use a hand mixer, and mix on medium speed until smooth.

3. Add icing mix and vanilla to the mix and mix on low.

4. Add heavy cream and mix on medium speed until thick.

5. Add melted chocolate to the mix and mix on medium.

6. Add mix to piping bag and pipe into cupcake tins, cover, and let them chill for at least 3 hours.

7. Serve and enjoy!

Per Serving Calories: 81 Fat: 8g Carbohydrates: 2.2g Protein: 1.8g

34 - Coco Popsicle

Preparation	Cooking	Servings
70 min	**0 min**	**8**

Ingredients

- 4 tablespoons cocoa powder, unsweetened
- 4 tablespoons chocolate chips, sugar-free
- 4 teaspoon natural sweetener
- 1 cup heavy whip cream

Direction

1. Blend the listed ingredients into your blender.

2. Blend until smooth.

3. Pour the mix into Popsicle molds.

4. Keep in the fridge for 2 hours.

5. Serve and enjoy!

Per Serving Calories: 210 Fat: 21g Carbohydrates: 4.2g Protein: 3g

VEGAN AND VEGETARIAN

35 - Garlic Aioli

Preparation	Cooking	Servings
15 min	0 min	4

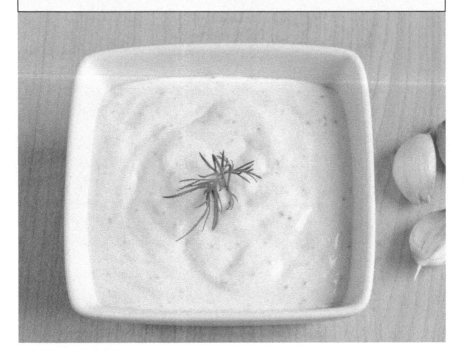

Ingredients

- 1 cup mayonnaise
- 4 garlic cloves, minced
- Juice of 2 lemon
- 2 tablespoon fresh-flat leaf Italian parsley, chopped
- 2 teaspoon chives, chopped
- Salt and pepper to taste

Direction

1. Add mayo, garlic, parsley, lemon juice, chives and season with salt and pepper
2. Blend until combined well
3. Pour into refrigerator and chill for 30 minutes
4. Serve and enjoy using Keto Friendly bread!

Per Serving Calories: 453 Fat: 68g Carbohydrates: 8g Protein: 2.2g

36 - Herbed Cream Cheese

Preparation	Cooking	Servings
15 min	**0 min**	**8**

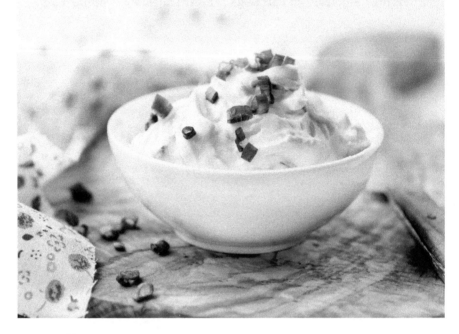

Ingredients

- 16 ounce cream cheese
- 4 teaspoons olive oil
- 1 cup fresh parsley, chopped
- 2 garlic clove
- 1 lemon, zest
- Salt and pepper to taste

Direction

1. Take a bowl and mix everything

2. Let it sit in fridge for 15 minutes

3. Serve and enjoy!

Per Serving Calories: 219 Fat: 75g Carbohydrates: 4g Protein: 3.2g

37 - Butter Mayo

Preparation	Cooking	Servings
15 min	2 min	4

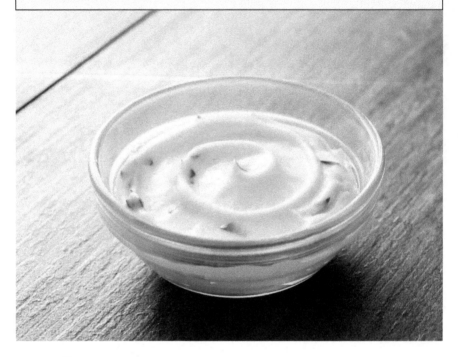

Ingredients

- 6 ounces butter
- 2 egg yolk
- 1 tablespoon Dijon mustard
- 1 teaspoon lemon juice
- ¼ teaspoon salt
- 1 pinch ground black pepper

Direction

1. Take a saucepan and melt butter
2. Pour into a small pitcher and let it cool
3. Take a bowl and mix in egg yolks and mustard
4. Pour butter into a thin stream and keep beating using hand mixer
5. Leave sediment at bottom
6. Keep beating until mixture thickens
7. Add lemon juice and season with salt and pepper
8. Use as needed!

Per Serving Calories: 245 Fat: 78g Carbohydrates: 0.8g Protein: 1.2g

38 - Spicy Wasabi Mayonnaise

Preparation	Cooking	Servings
15 min	0 min	4

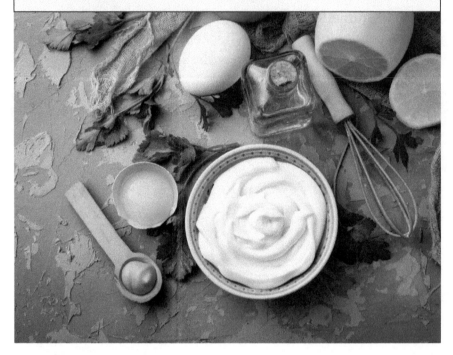

Ingredients

- 2 cup mayonnaise
- 1 tablespoon wasabi paste

Direction

1. Take a bowl and mix wasabi paste and mayonnaise
2. Mix well
3. Let it chill and use as needed

Per Serving Calories: 348 Fat: 41g Carbohydrates: 2g Protein: 2g

39 - Garlic Paprika Sauce

Preparation	Cooking	Servings
15 min	**7 min**	**8**

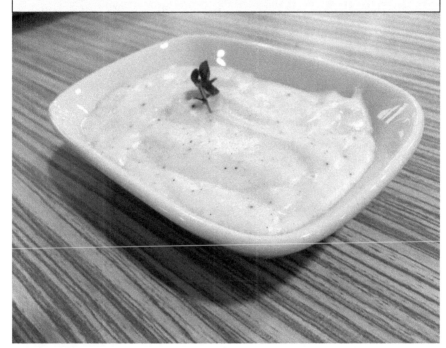

Ingredients

- 14 ounces butter
- 4 garlic cloves, chopped
- 2 scallion, chopped
- 2 tablespoon fresh chives, chopped
- 2 tablespoon fresh horseradish, grated
- 2 teaspoon dried thyme
- 2 teaspoon paprika powder
- 1 teaspoon salt
- 2 pinch cayenne pepper

Direction

1. Melt butter over medium heat in a saucepan
2. Add remaining ingredients
3. Whisk vigorously while simmer until sauce thickens
4. Serve and enjoy!

Per Serving Calories: 347 Fat: 31g Carbohydrates: 1.3g Protein: 1.4g

40 - Cashew Nuts Sauce

Preparation	Cooking	Servings
15 min	0 min	8

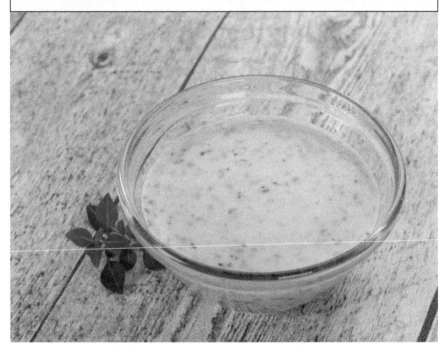

Ingredients

- 6 ounces cashew nuts
- 1 cup water
- 1 cup olive oil
- 2 tablespoons lemon juice
- 1 teaspoon onion powder
- 1 teaspoon salt
- 2 pinch cayenne pepper

Direction

1. Add nuts to your blender and process
2. Add other ingredients (except oil) and process until smooth
3. Add a little bit of oil and puree
4. Serve as needed!

Per Serving Calories: 341 Fat: 35g Carbohydrates: 5g Protein: 3.2g

REFRESHING DRINKS AND SMOOTHIES

41 – Baby Spinach Smoothie

Preparation	Cooking	Servings
10 min	0 min	4

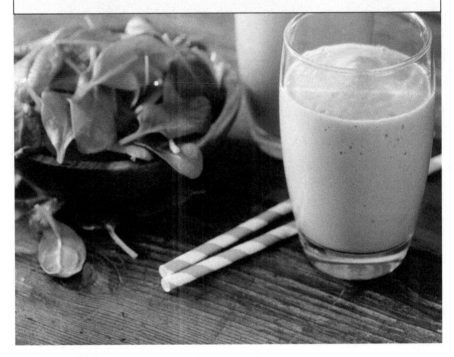

Ingredients

- 1 cup ice
- 4 cups baby spinach, chopped
- 1 cucumber, diced
- 1 cup frozen mango chunks
- 1 lime, juiced
- 1 lemon, juiced
- 2 cup of water

Directions

1. Add all the ingredients except vegetables/fruits first
2. Blend until smooth
3. Add the vegetable/fruits
4. Blend until smooth
5. Add a few ice cubes and serve the smoothie
6. Enjoy!

Per serving Calories: 113 Fat: 1.8g Carbohydrates: 14g Protein: 4.2g

42 - Kiwi Smoothie

Preparation	Cooking	Servings
10 min	**0 min**	**4**

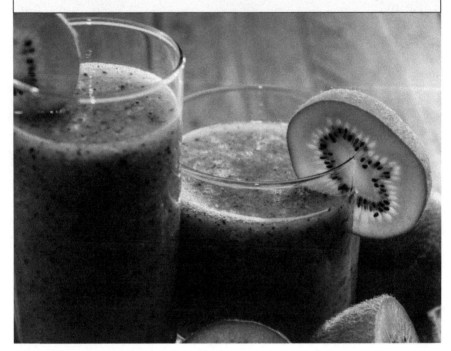

Ingredients

- 1 cup ice
- 2 cup baby spinach, chopped
- 1 cucumber, diced
- 4 kiwis, peeled
- 1/2 avocado, pit, and skin removed
- 2 scoop collagen protein powder
- 2 teaspoon freshly squeezed lime juice
- 2 cup of water

Directions

1. Add all the ingredients except vegetables/fruits first
2. Blend until smooth
3. Add the vegetable/fruits
4. Blend until smooth
5. Add a few ice cubes and serve the smoothie
6. Enjoy!

Per serving Calories: 228 Fat: 9g Carbohydrates: 13g Protein: 9g

43 - Mix of Papaya Smoothie

Preparation	Cooking	Servings
15 min	0 min	4

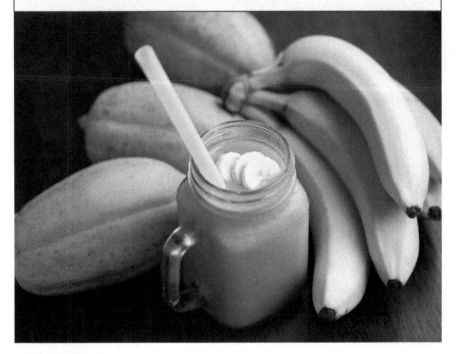

Ingredients

- 2 tablespoon hemp seeds
- 1 cup plain coconut yogurt
- 2 fresh banana
- 2 cup unsweetened coconut milk
- 3 cups frozen papaya blend (mix of papaya, mango, strawberry, and pineapple)

Directions

1. Add all the ingredients except vegetables/fruits first

2. Blend until smooth
3. Add the vegetable/fruits
4. Blend until smooth
5. Add a few ice cubes and serve the smoothie
6. Enjoy!

Per serving Calories: 176 Fat: 0.2g Carbohydrates: 12g Protein: 1.8g

44 - Mixed Berries Smoothie

Preparation	Cooking	Servings
10 min	0 min	4

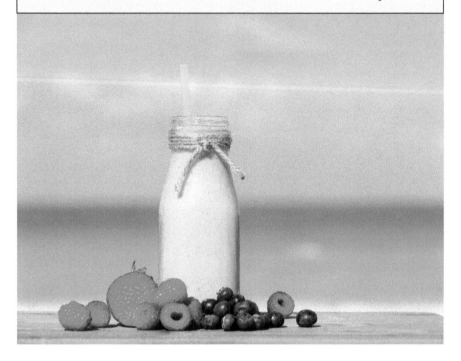

Ingredients

- 2 tablespoon chia seeds
- 1 cup of water
- 1 cup whole milk vanilla yogurt
- 2 cup frozen peaches
- 2 cup baby spinach
- 2 cup of frozen mixed berries
- 2 cup unsweetened vanilla almond milk

Directions

1. Add all the ingredients except vegetables/fruits first
2. Blend until smooth
3. Add the vegetable/fruits
4. Blend until smooth
5. Add a few ice cubes and serve the smoothie
6. Enjoy!

Per serving Calories: 157 Fat: 5g Carbohydrates: 16g Protein: 5g

45 - Strawberries Smoothies and Chia Seeds

Preparation	Cooking	Servings
10 min	**0 min**	**4**

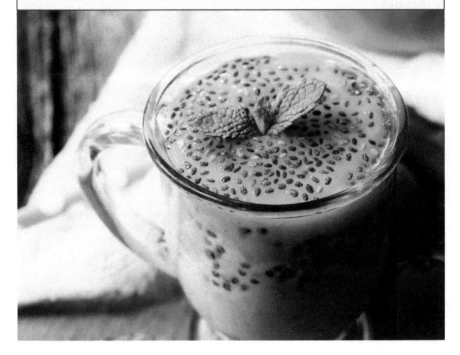

Ingredients

- 2 tablespoon chia seeds
- 2 clementine
- 1 cup plain low-fat Greek yogurt
- 2 cup of frozen strawberries
- 2 cup cantaloupe
- 2 cup unsweetened vanilla almond milk

Directions

1. Add all the ingredients except vegetables/fruits first

2. Blend until smooth
3. Add the vegetable/fruits
4. Blend until smooth
5. Add a few ice cubes and serve the smoothie
6. Enjoy!

Per serving Calories: 199 Fat: 3g Carbohydrates: 12g Protein: 11g

46 - Hearty Papaya Drink

Preparation	Cooking	Servings
10 min	0 min	4

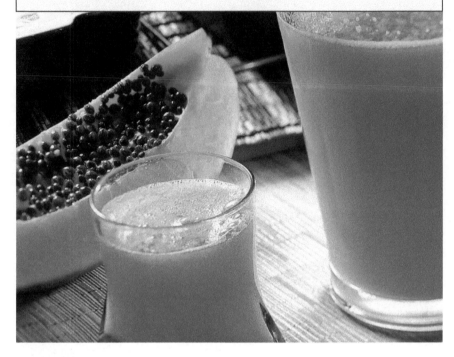

Ingredients

- 2 tablespoon chia seeds
- 2 cup plain coconut yogurt
- 2 cup baby spinach
- 2 cup frozen papaya
- 2 cup frozen tropical fruit mix
- 2 cup coconut milk, unsweetened

Directions

1. Add all the ingredients except vegetables/fruits first

2. Blend until smooth
3. Add the vegetable/fruits
4. Blend until smooth
5. Add a few ice cubes and serve the smoothie
6. Enjoy!

Per serving Calories: 182 Fat: 6g Carbohydrates: 14g Protein: 3.2g

47 - Fresh Minty Smoothie

Preparation	Cooking	Servings
10 min	0 min	4

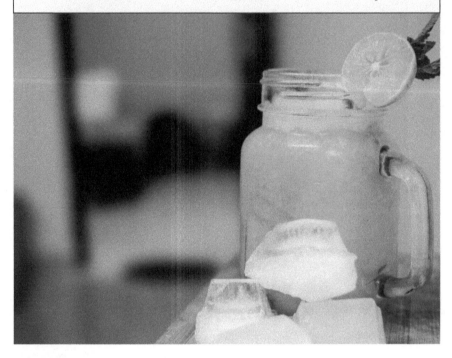

Ingredients

- 2 tablespoon hemp seeds
- Fresh mint leaves
- 1 cup plain coconut yogurt
- 2 cup of frozen mango
- 2 cup of frozen strawberries
- 2 cup unsweetened vanilla almond milk

Directions

1. Add all the ingredients except vegetables/fruits first

2. Blend until smooth
3. Add the vegetable/fruits
4. Blend until smooth
5. Add a few ice cubes and serve the smoothie
6. Enjoy!

Per serving Calories: 291 Fat: 9g Carbohydrates: 14g Protein: 4g

48 - Amazing Smoothie Acai

Preparation	Cooking	Servings
10 min	0 min	4

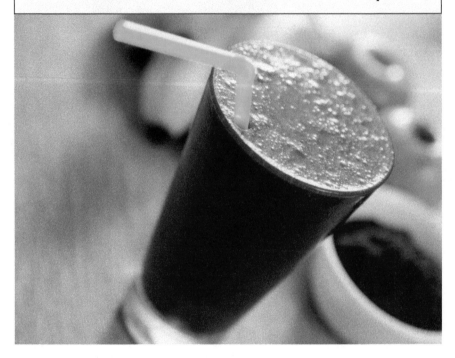

Ingredients

- 2 tablespoon hemp seeds
- 2 pack frozen acai
- 2 cup baby spinach
- 1 cup plain coconut yogurt
- 2 fresh banana
- 2 cup unsweetened hemp milk

Directions

1. Add all the ingredients except vegetables/fruits first

2. Blend until smooth
3. Add the vegetable/fruits
4. Blend until smooth
5. Add a few ice cubes and serve the smoothie
6. Enjoy!

Per serving Calories: 215 Fat: 7g Carbohydrates: 12g Protein: 4.1g

49 - Banana Matcha Smoothie

Preparation	Cooking	Servings
10 min	0 min	4

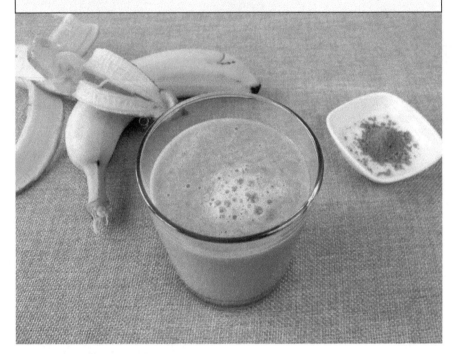

Ingredients

- 4 teaspoons matcha powder
- 2 tablespoon hemp seeds
- 1 cup of coconut yogurt
- 2 fresh banana
- 2 cup frozen pineapple
- 2 cup unsweetened almond milk

Directions

1. Add all the ingredients except vegetables/fruits first

2. Blend until smooth
3. Add the vegetable/fruits
4. Blend until smooth
5. Add a few ice cubes and serve the smoothie
6. Enjoy!

Per serving Calories: 216 Fat: 1.2g Carbohydrates: 14g Protein: 3.1g

50 - Green Garden Smoothie

Preparation	Cooking	Servings
10 min	0 min	4

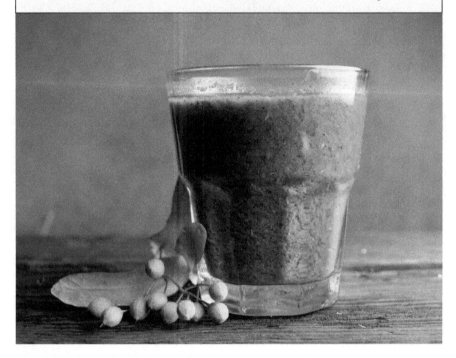

Ingredients

- 2 teaspoon spirulina
- Few fresh mint leaves
- 1 cup cucumber, peeled
- 1 cup plain coconut yogurt
- 2 cup pineapple, frozen
- 2 cup mango, frozen
- 2 cup unsweetened coconut milk

Directions

1. Add all the ingredients except vegetables/fruits first
2. Blend until smooth
3. Add the vegetable/fruits
4. Blend until smooth
5. Add a few ice cubes and serve the smoothie
6. Enjoy!

Per serving Calories: 210 Fat: 5g Carbohydrates: 14g Protein: 11g

Lightning Source UK Ltd.
Milton Keynes UK
UKHW020711270521
384463UK00001B/136